This Journal Belongs To

www.ingramcontent.com/pod-product-compliance
Lightning Source LLC
Chambersburg PA
CBHW072056280526
45788CB00006B/2308
* 9 7 8 1 0 9 3 4 0 1 2 6 4 *